BASIL

MARIAN KIM

ISBN: 1508550697

ISBN-13: 978-1508550693

CONTENTS

MARIAN KIM

1

PROPERTIES

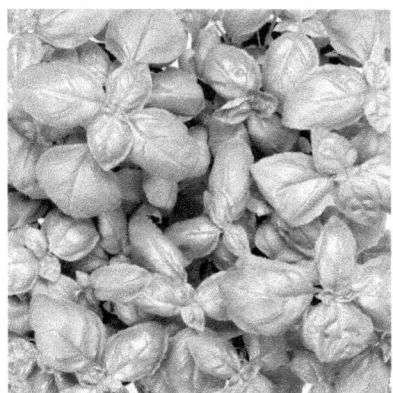

Scientific name: Ocimum basilicum

Other names: King of the herbs, tulsi, Saint Joseph's wort

Nutrients: Vitamins A, B9 (folate), C, K, calcium, copper, magnesium, potassium, iron, manganese, omega 3 fatty acids

Properties

The properties of basil include:

Anti-aging properties

Anti-cancer properties

Anti-inflammatory

Anti-oxidant properties

Antiseptic (antiviral and antibacterial) properties

Immune system boosting properties

Promotes hair growth

2

USES

Medically Proven Uses of Basil

High blood pressure treatment

Basil has been proven to lower blood pressure albeit temporarily.

***

Other Uses of Basil

Acne treatment

Basil is used for acne treatment because of its antibacterial properties.

Prematurely Aging Skin Management

Basil is used to prevent premature aging due to its anti-oxidant and anti-aging properties.

Lice treatment

Basil is used for lice treatment.

Thinning hair treatment

Basil is used to treat thinning hair and hair loss conditions since it improves the circulation of blood in the scalp and promotes hair growth.

Dandruff treatment

Basil is also used to treat dandruff and manage oily hair.

Depression management

Basil is used to treat depression due to its mood lifting properties and fragrantly sweet aroma.

Stress management

Basil is used for stress management since it acts a natural tranquilizer by calming the nervous system. Its powerful antioxidant properties are useful for helping the body cope with stressful situations when a lot of damaging free radicals are produced. 12 leaves of this adaptogen or anti-stress agent can therefore be chewed twice a day to prevent the effects of stress.

Headache treatment

Basil infusions (see recipe below) are used to treat headaches. The dried leaves can also be added to boiling water and the vapor inhaled to relieve headaches.

Coughs and colds treatment

Basil leaves act as expectorants and promote the removal of catarrhal and phlegm form the respiratory tract. They are therefore used to treat coughs, colds and bronchitis. Tea from the leaves can also be used to relieve sore throats.

Insect bite treatment

Basil is used to treat insect bites and stings. The juice from the leaves can be taken by mouth and applied on the insect bites to relieve the pain. Pounded fresh basil leaves can also be applied to the insect stings to possibly help draw out the venom. Basil is also used to treat snake bites.

Flatulence relief

Basil is used to manage digestive problems since it relieves flatulence or intestinal gas. The leaves can be steeped in water to make a tea that aids digestion. Basil is also used for stomach spasms.

Anorexia management

Basil is used to manage anorexia or loss of appetite.

Fever management

The juice of basil leaves works as an antipyretic and brings down the temperature especially in febrile children.

Wart treatment

Basil is used to treat warts.

Ringworm treatment

Basil juice is applied on ringworms to treat them.

Worm infestations treatment

Basil is used to treat worm infestations.

Birthing aid

Basil is used before and after childbirth to promote the circulation of blood in the pelvis and induce the flow of breast milk.

Halitosis treatment

Basil leaves can be boiled and the tea used as a gargle to manage halistosis or bad breath. The leaves can also be dried, powdered and mixed with oil to make toothpaste.

Mouth infections treatment

Basil leaves are chewed to treat mouth ulcers and infections.

Mental fatigue relief

Basil can relieve mental fatigue. It can also sharpen the memory.

Diabetes treatment

Some evidence suggests that basil tea or juice can stabilize blood sugar levels if drunk regularly.

Detoxification

Basil is also used for detoxification.

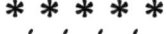

3

SAFETY PRECAUTIONS

None noted todate.

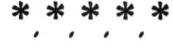

4

DRUG INTERACTIONS

None noted todate.

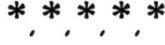

5

COOKING TIPS

Flavor: Fragrantly spicy

Goes well with: Tomatoes, poultry like chicken, Mediterranean cuisine like pizza, pesto, pasta and spaghetti sauce as well as salsas, shellfish, fish and cheese dishes.

Can be substituted with: Oregano or thyme or marjoram

Tips: Best used as whole leaves or if you must cut it, tear it at the last minute since the leaves can turn black. It should also be added to the dish at the last minute since cooking destroys its flavor. Smallest leaves are the sweetest. Thai basil has purplish stems.

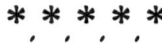

6

HERBAL RECIPES

Basil Infusion

Equipment

Glass jar with tight fitting lid

***

Ingredients

1 tablespoon dried basil or 3 tablespoons fresh basil

1 cup boiling water

***

Instructions

1. Place the herb in the glass jar and add the boiling water to fill the jar.

2. Close the lid and let the mixture steep for 4 hours to 14 hours (overnight).

3. Strain the herb and the infusion is ready for consumption.

***

Tips

1. Store the infusion in the refrigerator to lengthen its life.

*****

Basil Tincture

Equipment

Glass jar with tight fitting lid

Dark tincture bottles

Cheesecloth

Labels

***

Ingredients

7 oz (200 gm) of dried basil or 14 oz (400 gm) of fresh basil

30 oz (1 liter) of 80-100 vodka

***

Instructions

1. Fill 1/3 of the glass jar with the chopped basil.

2. Add the vodka to completely fill the jar to the top.

3. Seal the jar and label it with the date of preparation and name of herb used.

4. Store the glass jar in a dark place for 6 weeks ensuring that you shake it weekly.

5. After 6 weeks strain out the basil with a cheesecloth and pour the tincture into dark tincture bottles.

6. Label the tincture bottles with the date and name of herb used.

7. Store your herbal tinctures away from light and heat.

***

Tips

1. Pick your herbs early in the morning just after the dew has dried.

2. You can leave the herbs in the alcohol for up to 6 months if you want to create very strong tinctures.

3. To make your tinctures doubly strong, you can pour the tincture after straining in step 5 above and store it for six more weeks.

4. Though the dose varies, a standard dose is 1 teaspoon diluted in water or tea and taken 1-3 times a day.

*****

Basil Infused Oil

Equipment

Double boiler

Large glass bowl

Sieve and cheesecloth

Sterilized dark jars

***

Ingredients

16 fl oz. (500 ml) vegetable oils like sweet almond oil or sunflower oil.

8 oz. (250 grams) dry basil or 16 oz. (500 grams) fresh basil which is washed and slightly bruised.

***

Instructions

1. Place the basil and oil in the glass bowl ensuring that the oil covers the herb. Simmer them in a double boiler for one hour at a temperature of around 120 degrees Fahrenheit (49 degrees Celsius). Do not let the oil and herbs boil. You can repeat this step several times after letting the oils cool to create more concentrated herb infused oils. You can make your oils even more concentrated by adding a fresh bunch of basil with each re-simmering.

2. Strain the mixture through the sieve and cheesecloth into a clean, dark jar ensuring you squeeze out as much oil as you can from the herbs in the cheesecloth.

3. Label your jars with the manufacturing date, expiry date, herb and oils used.

4. Store your herb infused oils in a cool dark place or in the refrigerator and use them within 3 months.

*****

Basil Salve

Equipment

Double boiler

Large glass bowl

Sterilized dark jars or tins

***

Ingredients

8 oz. (250 ml or 1 cup) basil infused vegetable oil (see previous recipe)

1 oz. (30 grams) beeswax

10 drops essential oils like lavender essential oil

***

Instructions

1. Place the beeswax and basil infused oil in the glass bowl and melt them in a double boiler.

2. Once melted remove from the heat source and add the essential oils drop by drop.

3. Pour the melted oils into the storage jars or tins and allow them to cool completely.

4. Store the salves in a cool dark place.

***

Tip

If you want softer salves you can use less beeswax – for example ¾ oz of beeswax for 1 cup of basil infused oil.

*****

Basil Lip Balm

Equipment

Double boiler

Large glass bowl

Lip balm tubes or small jars or tins

***

Ingredients

3 tablespoons basil infused vegetable oil (see recipe above)

1 tablespoon grated beeswax

1 tablespoon shea butter

***

Instructions

1. Place the beeswax, shea butter and basil infused oil in the glass bowl and melt them in a double boiler.

2. Once melted remove from the heat source and pour into lip balm tubes allow to cool completely.

*****

Basil Butter

Equipment

Large glass bowl

Electric mixer or stick blender or wire whisk

Molds such as ice cube trays (optional)

***

Ingredients

½ cup butter

2 tablespoons of finely crushed, dried basil or 2 tablespoons of finely minced, fresh basil

***

Instructions

1. Place the butter in a warm place so that it can soften.

2. Put butter and your chosen herbs in a large glass bowl and blend well until thoroughly mixed.

3. Refrigerate until it hardens. You can refrigerate it in molds or ice cube trays to give it a special shape.

*****

Basil Tea

Equipment

Kettle

Tea cup

***

Ingredients

1 teaspoon of finely crushed dry basil or minced fresh basil

1 cup of water

Honey to taste

***

Instructions

1. Boil the water

2. Put the basil in a tea cup and add the boiling water. Let it steep while covered for 10 -15 minutes.

3. Add honey to suit your taste before drinking.

***

Tips

Basil tea can drunk for its healing effects or it can be added to a bath tub filled with warm water to aid with relaxation.

###

ABOUT THE AUTHOR

Marian Kim is an experienced alternative medicine practitioner.

*****

OTHER BOOKS BY THE AUTHOR

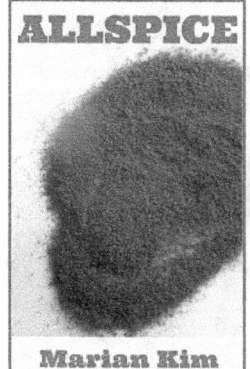

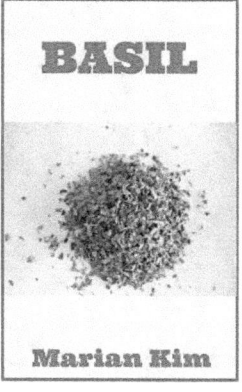

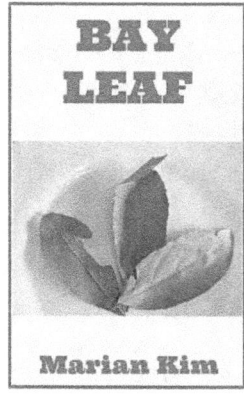

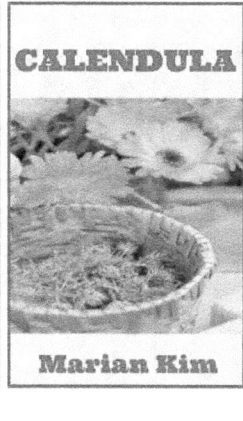

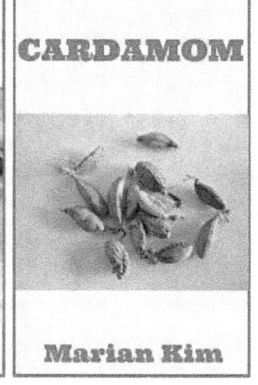

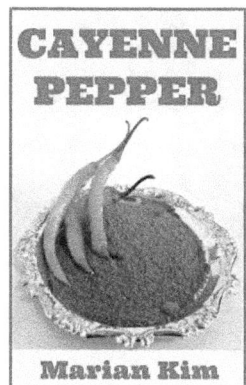

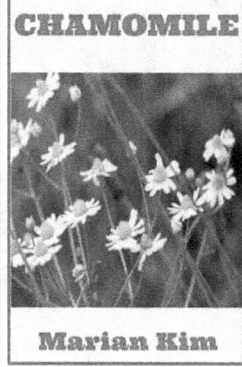

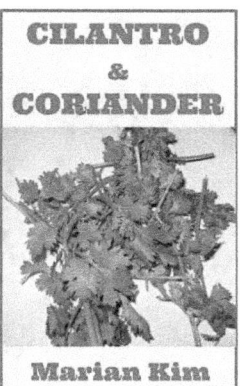

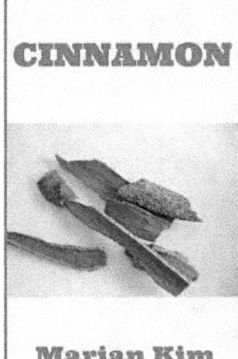
CINNAMON
Marian Kim

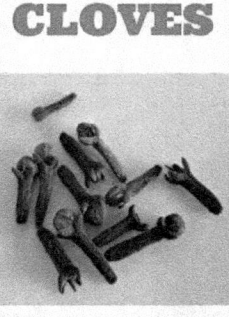
CLOVES
Marian Kim

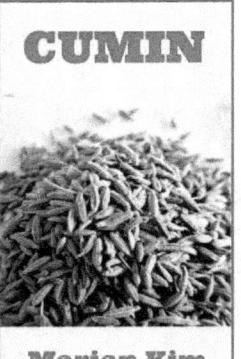
CUMIN
Marian Kim

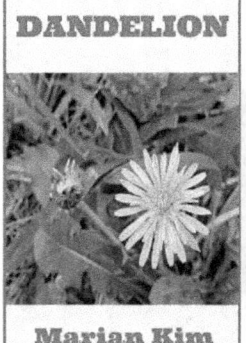
DANDELION
Marian Kim

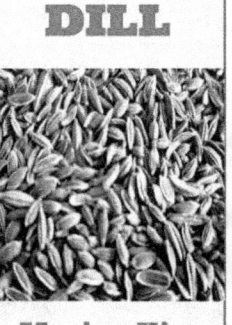
DILL
Marian Kim

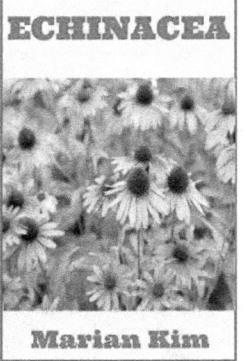
ECHINACEA
Marian Kim

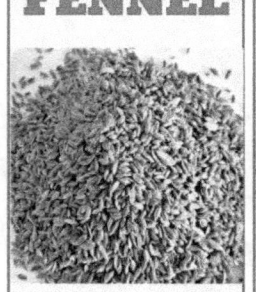
FENNEL
Marian Kim

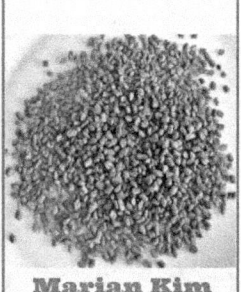
FENUGREEK
Marian Kim

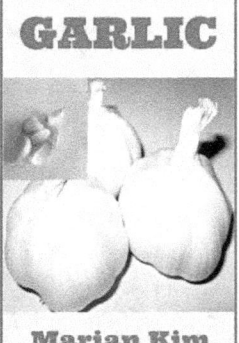
GARLIC
Marian Kim

GINGER

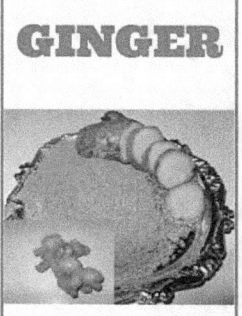

Marian Kim

GINKGO BILOBA

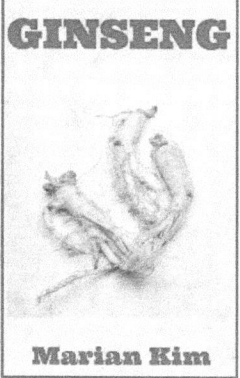

Marian Kim

GINSENG

Marian Kim

LAVENDER

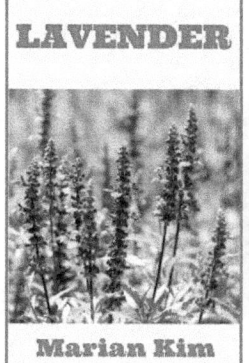

Marian Kim

MUSTARD

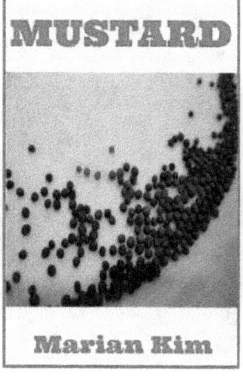

Marian Kim

NEEM

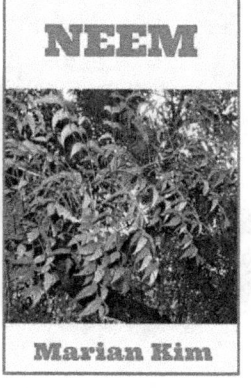

Marian Kim

NUTMEG & MACE

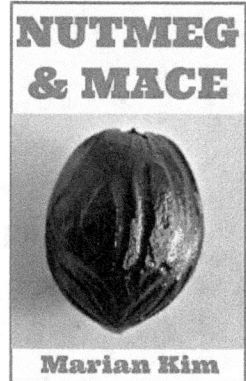

Marian Kim

OREGANO

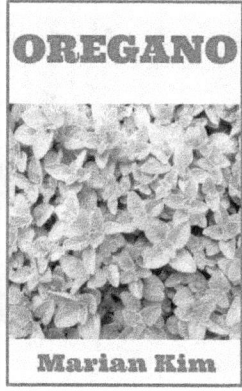

Marian Kim

PAPRIKA

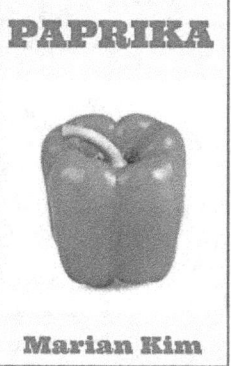

Marian Kim

PARSLEY

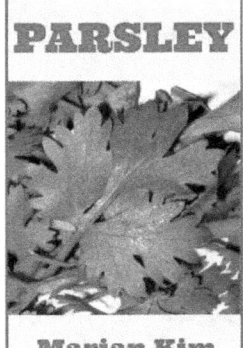

Marian Kim

BLACK & WHITE PEPPER

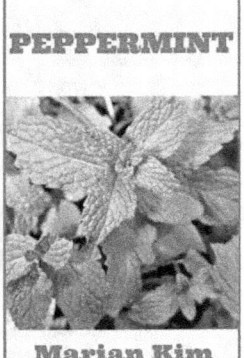

Marian Kim

PEPPERMINT

Marian Kim

ROSE HIPS

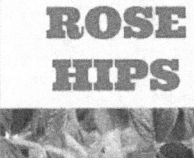
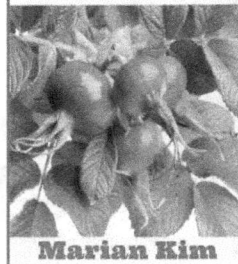

Marian Kim

ROSE PETALS

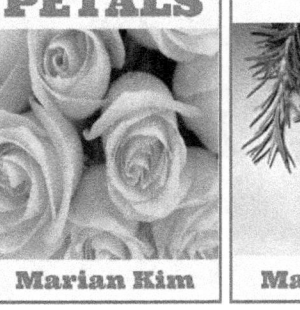

Marian Kim

ROSEMARY

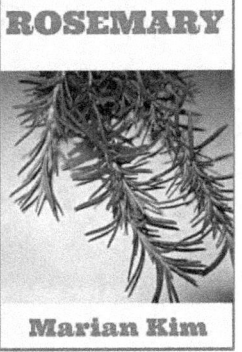

Marian Kim

SAGE

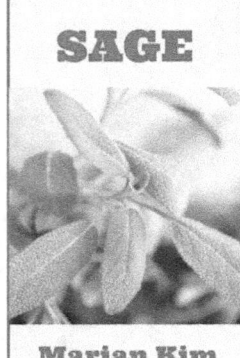

Marian Kim

ST. JOHN'S WORT

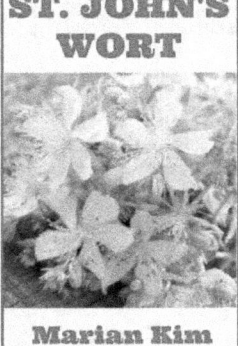

Marian Kim

STAR ANISE

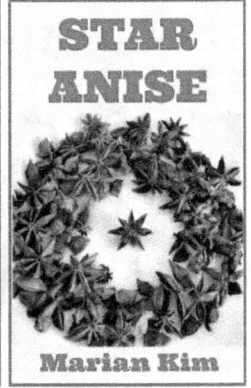

Marian Kim

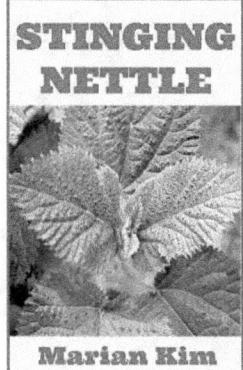

STINGING NETTLE
Marian Kim

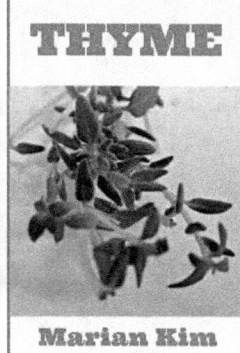

THYME
Marian Kim

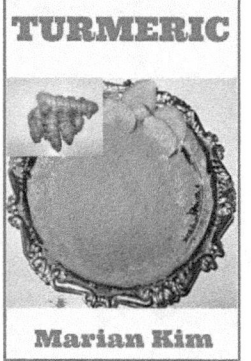

TURMERIC
Marian Kim

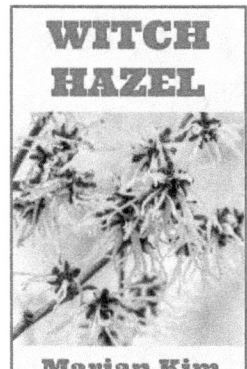

WITCH HAZEL
Marian Kim

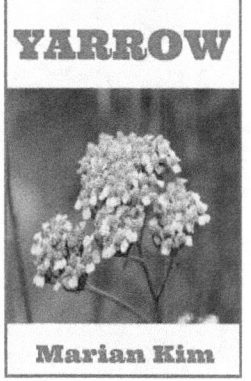

YARROW
Marian Kim

*****